Why The Swan Echoes?
I'm Just Saying

EVANGELIST MARY F. SIMMONS

Founder of Women of Faith and Power
Ministries, Inc.

http://womenoffaithandpowermi.injesus.com
womenoffaithandpower@yahoo.com

authorHOUSE®

AuthorHouse™
1663 Liberty Drive
Bloomington, IN 47403
www.authorhouse.com
Phone: 1-800-839-8640

First published by AuthorHouse 1/26/2010

ISBN: 978-1-4490-6168-5 (e)
ISBN: 978-1-4490-6167-8 (sc)

Printed in the United States of America
Bloomington, Indiana

This book is printed on acid-free paper.

Acknowledgements

If it had not been for the Lord who is always on my side, I would not have made it. He kept the wolves and all manner of evil from my door as I worked, researched, prayed, moaned and cried to finish this manuscript on time for His Glory and for my dedicated supporters.

Thanks be to the only Wise God my Saviour.

Contents

Not having grand children is not a blessing to me at all. I desire them more and more each day. My son Philip has never wanted children, which leaves a tremendous void in my life. He chooses older women to date or at least infertile ones. Why, I don't know for sure.

I dedicate this book to my Lord and Saviour Jesus Christ.

"Father, I thank you for all that you do for me, and that you allow me to do everyday of my life. I thank and praise you for your love and kindness to the children of men, and I pray that for each soul that reads this book, that they will will find you and serve you for the balance of their lives. In Jesus name.....Amen

Introduction

The Swan is a big beautiful bird with a voice as a trumpeter. Many years ago, I was attracted to this bird, or maybe not so much the bird, but what it stands for and portrays. This bird sings praises to God, its creator and maker. Man is created in the likeness and image of God, yet they have to be prodded and encouraged to praise the Lord, while this creature does not. What is wrong with this picture? I have often asked myself.

However, there are many different types of swans, I have chosen to bring "the black swan" to our attention in this book. The Black swan (cygnus atratus) is a large water bird which breeds mainly in the southeast and southwest regions of Australia. The black swan was first described by English naturalist John Latham in 1790. It was formerly placed into a monotypic genus chenopis.

The common name 'Swan" is a gender neutral term, however, 'cob' for a male and 'pen' for a female are also used as is "cyg (net" for the young. (1) collective nouns include a 'bank' (on the ground) and a 'wedge' (in flight). (2) black swans can be found singly, or in loose companies numbering into the hundreds or even thousands. (3) black swans are primarily black feathered birds, with white flight feathers. The bill is bright red, with a pale bar and tips, and legs and feet are greyish--black. Cobs (males) are slightly larger than pens (females) with a longer and straighter bill. Cygnets (immature birds) are a greyish--brown with pale--edged feathers. (4) A mature black swan measures between 110 and 142 cm (43-56 in.) in length and weighs 3.7--9kg (8.1-20 lbs). Its wing span is between 1.6 and 2 metres (5.3--6.5 ft.). The neck is long..............relatively the longest neck among the swans and curved in an "S."

The black swan is unlike any other Australian bird, although in poor light and at long range it maybe confused with a Magpie Goose in flight. However, the black swan can be distinguished by its much longer neck and slower wing beat.

God got down on His hands and knees, blew the breath of life into man and he became a living soul. Not the swan but man is made to be the praisers and trumpeter's for the Lord. The rocks will cry out, if human beings don't stand up and give the Lord the glory. It is not possible for a creature to take another's place in the presence of the Most Holy God. Life is most precious and sweet. Let us prepare to journey together as we discover why the swan echoes.

A few years ago, I was severally injured at physical therapy, when I was instructed to transfer all of my weight from the right leg to the left. In doing so, my left patellar tendon was ruptured, and it took seven surgeries as I endured infection after infection and a lengthy stay in the hospital and rehabilitation center to correct the problem. In the course of it all, the left knee was lost to the infection, therefore, I have no left knee. I walk with a limp and use a cane for support. My right knee is totally replaced, so you can imagine the rest of the story. Nevertheless, let me share my typical day with you. My day starts at eight in the mornings and end at eleven at night. During my first minutes of awakening I bless the Lord for allowing me to rest the previous night and for allowing me to wake up in the morning and we discuss what Ihope will be on my schedule for that day. Then, it is time to prepare for work, breakfast, ministry and whatever is thrown at me. Believe me, each day is a struggle. The angels are close to me, all of them...........to help me accomplish each and every task.

As a child I've believed in angels..........when my mother used to get sick or the babies would come in the middle of the night, it was me that my mother woke up to go and find my dad and let him know what was going on. The angels would accompany me and my dog Jack to the local speak easy to find dad, so he could go and get help. The road was long and dark back in the sixties growing up in Tillman South Carolina. There was no one else to depend on except the Lord and His angels. They camped around me and protected me from the wiles of the devil. The Lord has always protected me and He still does. Even as I journeyed to Philadelphia Pennsylvania, arriving there in the middle of the night on a greyhound bus, the Lord had prepared angels to come and deliver me safely to the place, where I was suppose to be. He has never failed me, nor do I expect Him to. I would always hear the saints say, there is no failure in God.....only beleive. In college my professor would say.....Have faith in God, if you can believe all things are possible because you believe. Faith is insurance with the only premium being confidence.

I have under went many different surgeries and procedures in my life with the aid of the Lord putting me in the hands of good capable angels such as doctors and nurses. Anyone can be an angel, that is why, we must be careful how we entertain strangers, because we entertain angels without knowing it. In my my daily life, I am aware of my darling angels. There are (1) ministering (2) fighting (3)waring (4) reaping (5) sowing (6) harvesting (7)comforting and (8) angels of light and please do not forget about our protecting angels.

These are the ones that I am sure of and of course, satan has transformed himself into an angel of light. We must know the differences between good angels and evil ones. The Lord uses each and everyone to help us to get through this life.

There has been many stories written about angels and how they have helped people in many different aspects of life. I am sure you have experienced aid from an angel. The question is: Did you thank your angel? We all have angels assigned to us. I believe it is important to get to know our angels personally.

Many times, as we are going through pain and suffering, we feel alone or maybe even lost, however, a noise or voice seems to come out of no where and startle us..........then we remember.....it must be my angel who came to encourage me. Often times the ministering angel will come singing a song or hymn, or maybe whistling a tune....you never know. We just have to create an atmosphere of peace and humility for the Lord and He will send an angel to comfort and care for you.

In my book "Sarah's Story", I tell of an angel that came to comfort little Sarah as she laid neglected in her crib, because her parents didn't want her due to her mental disability. The angels came and ministered to this little girl and taught her some wonderful things as she thrived all alone with love and care from her appointed guardian angel. Life became fulfilling for the little girl as she grew, and then one day, her mother heard her laughing and playing, and decided to go and see what was going on, and to her surprise it was af if Sarah had miracuously been healed. An angel brings good tidings from the Lord.

I. What's In your cup?

A cup can have bitterness mingled with sweet to disguise the pain and suffering that one will have to endure in life. The only thing you will experience as you drink it is........how good and freshing it tasted. Then all of a sudden it hits you. What have I drank? What was in that cup? Oh my Lord, what must I do? The answer comes...........this my child is what it is like to drink the cup of suffering. It doesn't seem like or it sure didn't taste like it, however, the pain is unbearable. Can you imagine this happening to you. Many times in life, we use drugs and alcohol along with bad dieting to our detriment, then it takes it toll on our bodies. Too much partying, fried foods, illicit sex, takes a toll on us as we age. The light begins to shine on us..........the big wake up call. The doctor brings the unkind news............cancer of the esophagus or some other type of cancer from over endulging. What am I going to do now, you may ask?

Weeping may endure for a night, but joy cometh in the morning. Once we realize, what we have done and to what extent the damage that has occured, a light begins to flicker and memory begins to sharpen. There is no danger in God's water, only that I have misused and abused this temple and I must pay. How great the price as we realize the years of stress and aggravation, self-denial that we have inflicted on ourselves, then comes the wake up call. Have no fear, you can began again and live your best life with some redirected knowledge and information. It will be costly and things will have to be given up and re-directed,

1

but through it all.............it will be worth it in the long run as long as the lesson is learned.

A voice we hear..........look up and live.   I will lift up mine eyes to the hills from whence cometh my help, all my help comes from the Lord.   I don't have to die, I must live and declare the works of my God. A glimmer of hope arises from the ashes, as we begin anew. The doctor enters the room, and begin to explain the procedure to get you back on the road to good health............surgery, chemo, radiation, therapeutic medications, rest, and dietary restrictions. Oh no doctor, one proclaims, I have another plan...........a master plan. What plan is that the doctor inquires? You see doctor, God designed this body and I messed it up by putting all the wrong things into it and doing all the wrong things with it, now I am going to realign my mind with the things of the Lord.   First, I am going to do a deep cleansing with herbs, fruits and vegetables while I pray and seek the face of the Lord. I will drink eight glasses of water a day, exercise and leave those fast people alone. Oh yeah, proclaims the doctor............ you will not be able to get better that way, becuase cancer has to be eradicated from the body by surgery followed by treatment and recoupment.   Well doctor, I will not do it your way, let me go back to the old land mark. The doctor walks out of the room and tells his staff, that man is dilutional with dementia, and we need to intervene on his behalf.

The doctor orders an injection of morphine to help with the pain, and the nurse enters the room to inject it through the intravenous tube, to find the patient up and dressed with the approratis removed from his vein. What do you think you are doing ask the nurse? I have came for my diagnosis replies the patient, now I am going to my healer.   Well I never said the nurse.   Well, I never been sick unto death either says the patient, now I am going to live and not die so I can proclaim the works of the Lord. The nurse had never experienced such behavior muchless a sure word from the Lord through a dying patient.   As he left the room, he took the nurse by her shoulders and told her, I will be healed by the stripes of Jesus, and when that happen he would come back and show himself.. The nurse's banner that day was "Well. I never".

II. Living your best life

The Holy Days of the Lord comes at different times of the year, yet most people take pride in calling them holidays. There is a vast difference in a Holy Day and a holiday. The difference is this: A Holy Day has been ordained and set aside by God with His presence injected therein. The Holy Days or Holy Convocations, Statutes are forever in our generations as long as we live. They are prescribed in the word of God. The Lord's Passover is a memorial of what the Lord did for us when he shed His blood on Calvary and the Days of Unleavened Bread commerates the deliverance of Israel and our deliverance from sin. Pentecost is a rememberance of when and how He sent His Holy Spirit to the churches, just as He promised by the mouth of Joel the Prophet. Feast of Trumpets is a memorial of blowing the trumpet which every knee will bow, every tongue will confess and every eye will see Him, and believe me, you will here the trump of God. The Day of Atonement..The Holiest Day of God's Calendar.........A rememberance for how God gave His only begotten son for you and I, because we could not atone for our own sins. It is a day for us to be at one with God. On this day we empty up all that we have done that has been wrong in the sight of God. Here is a list of things, that we don't even consider to be wrong and sinful. This is the day we afflict our souls for twenty four hours........evening unto evening...........no food, no drink. We confess and repent of: (1) weighty matters..........things that burden us down (2) sins that is committed because of greed, (3) sins of compulsion (4) gluttenous (5) medical neglect (6) emotinal blackmail (7)hardening our hearts (8) sins of unchasity (9) foreign unknown carnal knowledge (10) evil inclination (11) breaking the commandments (12) Incest (13) violence

(14) unjust scales (15) favoritism   (16) hypocrisy...... there are many other sins that are performed each day. As we repent of them, the Lord puts them far away from us, absolves, releases, annuls, makes them void and of none effect as long as we do not go back and practice them again. We must except the atonement of Jesus Christ to be fully justified and acquitted. Finally, the last and great feast............Feast of Harvest and Gathering......Sukkot. A time of sweetness and celebration, because we have made it right with God and there is nothing standing between of and our Savior.

The holidays cannot be compared with the Holy Days, because holidays are man made days and they do not glorify or magnify what the Lord has done for us. Holidays are just a figmentation of someone's imagination. As my siblings and I was growing up, our mother would say, they were just another day. These days are a good time for families to get together and most of the time it is all about food. Food has become for centuries the focal point of all cultures, large and small. I have come to the south to find that the festivals and each culture has different ways and customs to prepare and serve food. The Gullah community utilizes a lot of the bottom food................ creatures that feed off the bottom of lakes, rivers and oceans, which the Lord called scavengers. I believe this custom dates back to slavery. The Lord has a dietary law for His people. Eating of such foods eventually brings death. Hardship is something that one partakes such as pork products, and low bottom foods. Holidays ought to be about renewal and restoration, I do believe, not about loading up on unnecessary food.

Living ones best life has to do with lifestyle changes and our attitudes concerning life, and the pursuit of happiness. Joy is one of the components of the spirit, and it is much greater than happiness. Happiness depends on an happening, joy comes from the Lord and is permanent not temporarily. The family is another great asset for man and woman plus children. God designed the family to be a complete unit even for today. Let us embrace life as it was no tomorrow. Live your life and enjoy your life no matter the problem , you can do it, if you really have a desire. Put your best foot forward and march to the beat of a different drumer, there is no need to conform to this world or its standards. We are regal eagles. The eagle climb above the storms of life and soars to higher heights and deeper depths. Why just think about putting your feet and ankle in the water, why not your knees and waist, then get on your belly and swim to goodness and mercy. We must realize our dreams and goals, it is not just enough to have them, we must realize them in totality. Dr. Martin Luther King declared that he have a dream, not had a dream. Dreams are to be realized, lived, and it takeswork to bring them to fruition. It is no longer all right to be the best, we must be the greatest. Muhammid Ali, says he is the greatest, and during the thriller in Manila, he proved it. He and Joe Frazier were so tired each could hardly make it to their respectful corners, yet before the bell rang the greatest stood up and Frazier was intimidated, because he thought that

Muhammid Ali had recovered and there was no way that Frazier could compete with that, so he threw in t he towel by refusing to answer the bell. Will you be intimidated by the opponent in whimping out of your dreams. As I pass by all the cemetaries here in South Carolina, I am reminded of all the woulda, coulda, shoulda dreams that are stored in those graves. Don't let your dreams die with you. Dream big dreams................have lofty ideas and work hard to bring them to pass......ask the Lord to help you. I too have accomplished many dreams, yet, I have many more to accomplish. Let me share my accomplishments at the tender age of fifty-nine. The Lord has blessed me to be a published author, recording artist, a DVD of my early life, helper of others to bring their work into reality and I am still not finished. As the Lord prosper, we will be producing plays, writing more books, doing more recordings and helping us to write, produce or whatever the Lord allows. We have miles to go before we sleep. A little slumber and folding of the hands is all we need. Although, sometimes, our bodies requires more rest than sleep, so let us pace ourselves so we don't wear out before the day is done.

III. Alliances, Collaborations, & Partnerships

I believe it is important to build bridges that can and will take us across to the other side, because one never knows who will be over there once you have crossed. Alliances are unions that we form rather in marriage or work. These are so very important. God himself has formed an alliance with His people and it is up to us to sign on the dotted line. Having confidence in others will help to bring about prosperity and relationships in our lives. No one is successful all by themselves...........two are better than one, together they have a good report. Two heads are better than one, if one falls the other will be able to help the other up.

Collaborations simply means to work together in order to get the job done with mutual cooperation. Building a bridge takes cooperation, not working against one another. Many times we have to engage the help, expertise, or support from others to accomplish our dreams, visions or goals. Even Jesus, and we know that He is both God and man, yet He had to engage other's and still does to accomplish the great commission. Let's think about the empire's that has engaged others for duplication and productivity, such as food chains, clothing stores, herbal shoppes, auto dealerships and the like. No one is successful by themselves, we must have the help of others.

Partnerships are nothing new. There is nothing new under the sun, just some that we have not tried or humbled ourselves to do. The poor we will always have with us, simply due to the fact that we are too stubborn or big headed to ask. No one has all the answer, therefore, we have to build partnerships. Isn't it better to pull our resources together and purchase one pie or business or some other life changing idea than to sit around and live in poverty. Many nations of people pool their resources together in order to achieve success. It is important to practice what has been proven, there is no need to re-invent the wheel, when it has already been done. Learn how to plug into and ask for help. The reason why we have nothing is because we do not humble ourselves and ask for help. We must never give up........losers never win..............winners never lose....................presistence breaks down resistance. Let me share with you right here, right now some proven facts: . The Laws of Prosperity and Enrichment..........(1). The Ten Commandments of God is and must be the focal point that governs our entire being and lives everyday of our lives. The main goal now, will be spiritual and not material. It will follow your walk with God and live by every word that comes from the mouth of God.......Your education and entire preparedness wil be different. You will seek to learn the true values of life............yes, this life and the life to come. The health of everyone you care about will be important to you beginning with your spiritual, dietary, emotional, physical, psychological, cultural and social. We will think different, therefore our thoughts and actions will reveal it in our contenance. (2). Certainly nothing in life is more relevant than to realize what is real success and how to achieve it. Establish your goal or dream, vision in writing, because it is a proven fact, that people who record their hopes and dreams on paper will achieve them. It will give you a road map to follow and help with your journey into prosperity and wealth. Just as it is important to sow that right seed, it is also important to fix the right goal...............not just any goal..............one plant, another water, and the increase comes from the Lord......Speak to other like minded people about your dreams, goals and visions. The right goal includes something more. We must be able to define success!   Once we have learned what success is we must be able to make that your goal. What we think about the most, will become ours. It is important to study success from every angel, and the lives and lifestyles of successful people. I am not talking about money alone, but everything that causes a person to be successful. The Lord has a plan and a purpose for our lives, for us to prosper and not to harm us, however, few inquire of God......what that plan is and how to accomplish it. (3). Preparation to achieve that goal is vital.   Read and listen to everything that you can find that speaks to this subject. This is called educating one's self ...knowledge is powerful. Don't allow your emotions to control you here.   A friend of mine attended a seminar, and during the presentation, she was overwhelmed with all the details, so she fell asleep. Upon awakening, the presenter was standing over her and asking her, if she had made a decision concerning the product.   She smiled and said, you know what, I like the way you look, sound and handle yourself, therefore, I will join your group.   That was a bad idea, because, first of all, she had no prior knowledge of the product, and neither had she heard all the information. This was like whipping a dead horse. She went to the bank and withdrew all of her money and bought the product and a year later she was dead broke and still holding a product that was untaped because she refused to gain the necessary knowledge in order to market the product. We are not to get involved with things on a feeling or a whim. (4). Excellent Health is nothing to sneeze at...it is the key to realizing and accomplishing our dreams. Earlier, we spoke of alliances, partnerships, collaborations in order to be able to carry out our great commissions. These can and will play an important role if you are not in good health.......on the other hand, why would you want to start a business or venture if you are not able. Think about it...........the presence and expert wisdom is detrimental especially in the formable years. Of course there are many things that can rob us of our health.............lack of sleep and rest, excess alcohol, drugs, salt, fats, sugar, tobacco, going against the dietary laws and the lack of exercise. One of the key ingredients after you have educated yourself on your chosen goal is to have a complete physical to ensure you can at least from a medical stand point go the distance. One of the greatest mistakes we sometimes make as we start a new business is not to train someone to assist us and be able to carry on in the event life presents some challenges. A wise person never leaves nothing to chance. (5). Insurance is the next key in this process. Life, health, disability and worker's compensation as well as business insurance to cover those unfore seen emergencies. A cup of prevention is worth a cup of cure. (6). An inactive person will not be able to go the distance.............faith without works is dead.......... we must work. Any dead fish can swim down stream, it takes a live one to swim up stream................and inactive person will not accomplishment anything. I often get referred to by my staff and friends as a trane...........can you stop a trane? No you can't, that is why I stay alert

with an excellent spirit and a good atitude.   Very little
get me down,,,,,,,,,,,,,,My focus is on being a tramp for
the Lord and pleasing Him, therefore, I know, I cannot
please Him if I am tired and worn out from eating all
the wrong foods, no exercise, and a bad attitude, no one
would want to be around me, muchless work with me.
We must stay prayerful and focus at all times. (7). All
has been achieved, checked and tripled check................
training, educated, experienced in pursuing, kept in good
health, and constantly driving yourself relentlessly toward
your objective, that you would accomplish your dream.
Important as these principles are, they are not enough.
Life constantly encounters hazards, obstacles, unexpected
problems or setbacks. We may be proceeding along right
on schedule, then bang!............out of nowhere comes an
unexpected complication. Some unexpected circumstance
arises which seems to stop us completely, or at least set us
back. Subsequently, we must be equipped with resources.
Resourcefulness to solve the problem, overcome the
obstacle, and stay the course. This is why you will have
incorporated an expanded relationship with the Lord, so
we can call on Him and He will send help to our aid, and
have a data base of people to rely on. There must not be
left one stone that is unturned. Should there be a dead
cow on the tracks...............it will bring everything to a halt
until the corpse is removed.

Finally, perserverance is the key that locks the door
to our success............stick......to........it.......ness.   Failure
is not an option..............you have prepared yourself to
be a winner.................bonapetit.............congratulations
success has arrived.

IV. Friendship

Friendship with Jesus............what a fellowship divine. Life is full of surprises, nevertheless, this great union is undisputed. Flowers bloom and fade........................ friendship never diminshes where there is love and compassion one to another. It is a treasure to be protected...............a fine wine to be enjoyed............a long walk in the woods with so many different things to see and experience. A friend loves at all times and does not sympathize with my weaknesses or failures, yet finds empathy to help me through my losses and ensures me how to find prosperity and contentment in the victory to be won on tomorrow. Penquins are friends to each other, this is personified in their mannerism, behavior and attitude None is left behind while the fox sits on the bank of the river waiting for them to forsake their code of honor.

Did you know you were courageous, strong and in control. Did you know there was one watching as you picked up your friend after banadging her wound, placed her in your arms and took her to the emergency room. Did you know that someone prayed for your strength and her recovery. Did you know how much you encouraged others to do the same. Did you know someone who was watching found grace to carry on. Did you know my heart was touched and changed, just because of your love and kindness.

Good friends are like a nice warm cup of tea, it soothes one's soul. A good friend is like the sun setting, it will rise in the morning.   It is like a cake in the mixer, there surely will be some batter left to taste.   Oh taste and see, for the Lord is good.   I thank God for your rememberance.   My friend speaks to me, talks and walks with me, comforts me and encourages my heart. She is never to busy to listen.   She never reminds me of my faults, she covers them with love.   She walks by my side even when things are not well with her.   Her love is steadfast and unmoveable.   She believes all things and loveliness surrounds her with gold.

We love each other deeply and no one can separate us from the love of God.   A true friend is a precious gift that God has placed in the life of this earthen vessel to be a blessing.   Although, I realize and she knows how deeply we have hurt each other, forgiveness and healing has erased all rememberance for we have moved on to perfection.   Laughter and praise is the banner we wear because the blood of Jesus has removed all stain.   There is no need or desire to look back because all has been forgiven..........all that is left is to keep the faith, finish our course in victory.

Did you know my friend, this is all that is required of us. Oh yes, one more thing.............Lord help my friend to endure hardness as a good soldier, as she prepares for battle.   Today, I claim victory over her by putting the whole armour of Yahweh upon her life. I place the girdle of truth upon her heart, may she stand firm in the truth of God's word with the helmet of faith and the breast plate of righteousness...............your love means everything to me..............here I am standing with my heart and arms open waiting for your return.

V. Losing Control

Let your moderation be known unto all men. Naked we came into this world and naked will we leave at least the physical. Our life ought to be an open book, nothing hiding. Our control and guard ought to be intact especially if we say that we have been changed and redeemed by the shed blood of Jesus. Honesty is the foundation of change. There is nothing to hide, the covers is off just as it was in the garden of eden before Adam and Eve sinned. No longer ashame to testify of wrongs knowing that we overcame by the word of our testimony and the blood of the lamb. There is now no condemnation to those that are in Christ Jesus. Everything about us is covered in and under the blood of Jesus, and we have surrended all to Him, therefore, we fear not what man can do to us. Boldness has become our banner and shield. My garments are truth, honesty, just, love, purity, a good report, virtue, praise and holiness.

VI. Astonishingly Familiar

There was something astonishing familiar in her tone. The swan echoe reigns in the upcoming summit. She has been predicting snow for the Carolina's frequently. Traveler's are venturing from the north not knowing the forecast ahead predicts snowy days and balmy nights. The South is becoming more northernly with everyone migrating south. Prosperity the horizon again, because there are no differences between the regions. Our languages are distinct with multiple dialects such as, gullah, creole and geechee. It reminds me of Pentecost, as everyone recognized their own native tongue. For the life of me, it is difficult to understand geechee. Everyday dress and culture blends easily and northern visitors embrace it like a duck taking to water or a possum to the swamps as it wets our appetite for a little snow and ice. It would be nice to have a snow festival here south of broad.

Life is so exciting and it seems to me the older I become the more resonation suits me. Fire side chats, off beaten plays, real butter on my bread dripping with warm maple syrup, kick your shoes off, cuddling, rubbing noses together like the eskimos, long walks in the woods, horse back riding, fox trots, calf herding and wrestling, cider sipping, hop scotch and hayrides and a little down home hoot nannie..........yippie do da........getti up cowboys and girls. I hear my swan echoing............come out and play with me.

Old ancient relics encased in museums with over sized paintings that belong in spooky mansions. We enjoy older men with white beards, neatly cropped of course with a dapper daddy walk imitating John Wayne and moves like Elvis Presley. We like the old gospel and blues mixed with a healthy heaping of southern jazz with a side of grits and fish with mustard and hot sauce.

Favorite smells reminds me of Grandma's home cooking with a finger of love stuck in the middle. The swan echoes, with every whisper of real coconut pies, made from whole grainh bread that is baked to perfection and served with fresh butter milk. Fruit cake with all fresh nuts, hand picked and craved at its peak of sweetness, carefully crafted into a mixture, with all ingredients, placed carefully in baking dishes.

Many days I think of the hundreds of people that I've had the opportunity to interview and speak with concerning the things that they remember or even go through in their lives. Some tell of evil influences and how the devil afflicts their bodies with incurable diseases. Others of being manipulated, emotional black mailed and even drugged into submission. One lady related her story to me in this manner: I met a man and he convinced me that he was the only man for me, through manipulation, manopolizing all of my time. In other words each time she looked around, he was there trying to influence her every decision. He went as far as to alienate her from family and friends. The devil is as a roaring lion, seeking whom he may devour. He is not a lion, he just acts as if he is........to get you upset and confused, so you will make rash decisions. This particular woman, went on to say, he convinced her that she was a burden to her family and they had asked him to marry her so she would have someone to take care of her. This was a very wealthy and secure woman before she allowed this man to influence her life and decisions. Once the devil has control over you, he wants to take over and control everything that you have.

In my audio book "Set the captives free", I explain many different ways as to how the evil one can come and steal your mind, thoughts, ideas and even your future, yet, there are ways to safe guard against all the works of darkness today and forever. Even sometimes, your friends and families will conspire against you because of jealousy, envy and other manners of evil. We must always keep our minds on the Lord and He will keep us in perfect peace. I love the 37th Psalm..............it reminds us not to fret ourselves because of evil doers. Women are not the only ones that fall prey to works of darkness. Men can be easily influenced by wicked devices, and cunning women. This is why we must stay prayerful, focus and in the word of God. Our minds must be stayed upon the Lord and not leaning to our own wondering thoughts and ideas. We must know our core self..............leave nothing to chance. Do not leave yourself open and vunerable, especially when you are not feeling good about yourself. Low self esteem is the enemy's play ground. Build yourself up in the Lord. Never leave home without first spending time in the word and prayer............nothing else will sustain you...........nothing.

The swan echoes for many different reason, however, the greatest is for those who will not, desire not, have not the mind to or refuse to praise the Lord. It only takes a few minutes to give thanks................Oh that the children of men would give thanks. Many have and are without hope, yet the Lord is your hope, only receive Him today and turn not away.   Find hope in Jesus Christ, a hymn, song, poem, poetry or even a bird singing.   Today, when you hear His voice, do not harden your heart.

Time and chance happens to us all.   The question is not if........it is when.   The storms of life is raging, yet the Lord is standing with His arms stretched out, waiting for you to walk in and believe me, He will in no wise cast you out.   Don't allow the enemy to keep you upset and confuse................Christ is the answer, and He has all the answers.

VII. We teach others how to treat us.

It is important to watch our actions as well as the signals we present.   Our attitudes speaks louder than words we speak.   Someone is always watching and observing our every move, rather we know it or not.   My former Pastor would always assure me, everytime you speak, move, laugh or breathe, remember someone is watching you, so be careful and aware of your actions. The way we behave in public does affect others, somebody wants to be like you and they will imitate your behavior. Every time I stand to speak, teach, preach or even testify, I am training someone. Psalm 37........instructs us to mark the perfect and upright man, for at the end of that man or woman is peace.

Who are you marking or setting an example for?   It has been said, the chip doesn't fall far from the tree.   In my young life, I wanted to emulate my Pastor..............Rev. Rance Youmans.   Why, because, he could preach like no other and imitate I did.   After church, I would go home, change my clothes and preach to whatever or whomever was around.   My grandparents and aunts would get a kick out of me, and even until this day, I have studied and prepared to be a great teacher and preacher and I know that I come second to none. Yes, I am bragging, yet not of myself, rather of my Lord. He gave me this excellent gift in this earthen vessel. I live to preach and teach the gospel..............if you think that I am not serious about the work of the Lord just invite me to speak at your church or worship center. I have been anointed to preach the gospel and to heal the broken hearted.

Carry yourself in a dignified manner with all authority and power that the Lord has given you. Do not act like a target or one with low self esteem. Hold your head high and if you are not feeling it, please act if you do. We are the head and not the tail, above only and not beneath. Winners never lose, and we have a lot to look forward to. God has placed us here to be His joy and helper. Let the your words be yea and nay. Mean what you say, and own it all the time. It does not matter what you wear as far as clothes is concerned, just let them be clean and pressed. Walk with dignity and be full of integrity. It does not matter where you live or where you have been. You may live in the ghetto, it does not mean the ghetto is in you. Build yourself up with positive information. Look in the mirror and tell yourself, I am God's favorite child, no matter where I roam it belongs to me. I look good, smell good, feel good, therefore, I will do great and have mighty things to day. Feed yourself good and positive information. When people pay you a compliment, thank them with a big smile and say to yourself..............I know that. Hold your head high, because you are God's highly favored child and He has given you preferential treatment. People will respect you, open doors for you, and give you opportunities that you haven't even earned. Walk and act like a millionare and you will become one. Dream faith dreams, have a plan of action and talk of them often. It does not matter rather people will support you or not...........say the word, believe and you shall receive. As your friends and family begin to see, they will be jealous and envious.......let them, you just keep on doing your thing and God will bless you to do more. Don't allow pride to slip in or your feet to slip into their way of thinking. Say it, be it, do it and own it! Life is too short to keep looking back. Live and think prosperity.

VIII. Life is not cured, just managed.

Successful keys to managing life are: 1. You are your own life manager, no one can manage your life for you. Not your family, friends, doctor, minister or even the Lord. They are there to provide information, support, love and guidance, it is up to you how to proceed. 2. Foolishly risking your life's savings on frivolous things. 3. Learn to utilize all your skills and abilities. 4. Maintain your health and well being, spirit, emotions, financial, psychological, physical, medical, social as well as cultural. 5. Healthy relationships and your well being free from abuses of all types allows you to prosper and flourish. 6. Are you reaching and stretching for those things that will keep you fresh, young, and alive? 7. Design your day-to-day so it will flow with your style................ so you enjoy some relaxation, peace and tranquility. 8. Arranging for some fun and recreation in your life will allow you to dream of creativity. 9. Structuring your world so that there is balance among these things you to be important.

As long as we're alive, there will never be a day when every single one of our problems has been wiped clean. Some days will, of course, be dramatically better than others. In the end, it is up to us to build and enjoy those particular days. We must learn how to be an effective "life manager." Work toward resolving, rather than enduring all of life's cares. Draft realistic expectations rather than naive ones. Learn to regard success as an always

-moving target. Without a conscious, well considered strategy, more than not that success will not allude us if we perservere and be persistent.

There are many people who think others are responsible for their existence, let me assure you that this is the farthest thing from the truth. The government, state agencies, non profits or no organization is responsible for our well being it is up to us to figure it out for ourselves. The world does not owe us nothing. Many of our fore parents laid the foundation, but it took God to open up the way. We must get up off of the couches, bathe, comb our hair, get dressed and go out and make it happen. I would like to give you a fish so you can enjoy a meal today, nevertheless, I will teach you a trade, like fishing so you can feed yourself for a life time. It is our life, it is up to us to manage it everyday.

Laziness is one of the down fall of our people. We cannot be lazy and prosper. The Lord instructs us if we do not work then we ought not to eat! How shocking, you might say.....well, I say Amen.....Amen. Even people with disabilities earn degrees, work and care for themselves and their families. Creativity is a great way to do many things. A few years ago, I ruptured my patellar tendon in the left knee. After under going seven surgeries it was not looking good for me to ever walk again muchless work at my craft. The doctors was not hopeful at all, yet, my faith, support and encouragement from my family and friends kept me going. A few days after the third surgery, the doctors ran more test and assured me that I would in all probability lose my artifical left knee because of the infection. Yes, I did, but I did not concentrate on my disability, rather my ability. Oh course, I had to reprogram my mind and brain to focus on what I had, not what I had lost. The Lord had and has blessed me to have more than enough to begin again. Today, I walk with the use of a cane, write, publish, travel and spend time supporting others at Penn Center. My most important tool is my excellent spirit and positive attitude. Utilizing these tools have opened many doors for me and they will take me before Kings and Queens and allow me to witness to great and small.

Therefore, let us refocus our tools, change our attitudes from negative to positive and allow the Lord to bring out of us what He intended from the beginning. There are so many that have failed more than once, some many times, yet they did not give up, rather they redirected their wealth, knowledge and resources and began again. Take a little time out and do some research on our founding father's and mother's who have paved the way for us. Don't focus on your past mistakes.............your past does not equal your future. Your future can and will be redirected if you will only put the right information in your mind and spirit. All things are possible if you can only believe.

We have to envision our future...............".without a vision, people perish".What is your vision? Write it down....it has been proven, people who write down their vision obtain more success than those who don't. "Change is one of the most difficult things in the world, yet, those who embrace change never complains." We do what works for us! How about allowing change to embrace you, first with the way you think or walk even travel, the company you keep. Birds of a feather flocks together..........who are the birds you are flocking with and what are you doing with them that is so important it is keeping you from your dreams and goals? Let me challenge you right here right now to examine your motives for pursuing this line of action.

If the grass is greener on the other side...........Earl Nightingale writes: It's probably getting better care. Success as a human being is not a matter of luck (prepardeness meets and opportunity) or circumstances. It's not a matter of fate or the breaks you get or who you know. Success is a matter of sticking to a set of common sense principles anyone can master. The magic word in life is "ATTITUDE". It determines our actions, as well as the actions of others. It tells the world what you expect from it in return. As you accept responsibility for your attitude, you accept responsibility for your entire life. It is just as simple as that! We cannot change what we do not acknowledge.

IX. The swan says, portray all these

1. Honesty-----------the foundation of change
2. Openmindedness----accessible to new things and ideas, enlightened
3. Gratitude------------Thankfulness
4. Responsibility-----Taking Ownership of One's Action
5. Caring---------Showing Compassion & Empathy
6. Humility-------------humbleness, meekness
7. Objectivitity-------------fair, impartial
8. Willingness-----readiness to accept or under take

Portrayal is an attribute to be designed, embraced and applauded. Have you ever heard of wearing your feelings on your sleeve? Well it is not your sleeve that concerns me, it is your facial expressions. I can along with many other people tell what you are feeling, simply by watching your expressions or lack thereof. Bad times are inherent, it will happen, but the most important rule is to control our emotions. Leave the resentments at home, check them at the closing of the door. No one wants to deal with bad behavior muchless ugly behavior. The higher one goes in an organization, the better the attitude. One of the things I pray about each mornings is peace. Follow peace with all men, holiness without no man shall see the Lord. Let me assure you,without a good attitude no one shall see wealth and prosperity in their lives. We have no one to blame for our lack of a good attitude, the ability to wear a smile or to give a pleasing smile. Another way to have favor is to remember names, special occassions and to compliment others especially those we love and need to help us through life. " No man or woman is an island to themselve's." People need people to get through life.

As I travel through the cities, states and other regions, my main focus is to "do unto others as I would have them do unto me", with love, understanding and compassion. It all comes from my heart, if I don't mean it, I won't say it or do it. And this applies to praying for people and giving them a word of prophecy. Life is to important for me to be a

phony or pretender. People need and want realness, so lets practice it and give it freely.

"Like a city whose walls are broken down is a man who lacks self-control," Proverb 25:28. He is defenseless and doomed to defeat.

"Be the change you wish to see in the world."----- Gandhi

"To thine ownself be true."

"Own what you are."

"Celebrate your beauty and greatness."

Stay the course to your dreams, yes, you may stumble even fall down--------rise again, dust yourself off and start again. Don't allow the nay sayers to influence you............. always wear a smile with an excellent spirit.

X. Poems and Sayings

Standing Alone

One night as I sat looking out the window I saw a
shawdow standing alone.
Alone as if nothing else mattered at all. We stand alone
more often
than we can imagine, even while in a crowded room.
Loneliness is an epidemic in these United States and around
the world...............Evangelist Mary F. Simmons

Beginning The Day

I got up early one morning and rushed right into the day,
I had so much to accomplish that I didn't have time to pray.
Problems just tumbled about me, and heavier came each
task.
"Why doesn't God help me?"
I wondered, He answered,
"You didn't ask"
I wanted to see joy and beauty,
But the day toiled on, gray and bleak;
I wondered why God didn't show me. He said,
"But you didn't seek!!"
I tried to come into God's presence,
I tried all my keys at the lock.
God gently and lovingly chided
"My child you didn't knock,"
I woke up early this morning and
paused before entering the day;
I had so much to accomplish that I had
to take time to pray.

BLACK FAMILY PLEDGE

BECAUSE WE HAVE FORGOTTEN OUR
ANCESTORS,
OUR CHILDREN NO LONGER GIVE US
HONOR.
BECAUSE WE HAVE LOST THE PATH OUR
ANCESTORS
CLEARED, KNEELING IN PERILOUS
UNDERGROWTH,

----DR. MAYA ANGELOU-----

Little Jelly Beans

Little jelly beans
Tell a story true
A tale of our Father's love
Just for me and you
GREEN is for the waving palms
BLUE for the skies above
BROWN for the soft earth where
People sat hearing of HIS love.
A SPECKLED bean for fish and sand
RED for precious wine
And BLACK is for the sin He washed
From your soul and mine.
PURPLE'S FOR THE SADNESS OF
HIS family and friends,
And WHITE is for the glory of the
Day HE rose again.
Now you've heard the story
You know what each color means
The story of our Father's love
Told by some jelly beans.
So every morning take a bean
They're really very yummy
Something for the soul, you see.
And something for the tummy.

One afternoon as I sat in my office, a beautiful woman walked in, dressed in red from her head to toe, and presented me with some jelly beans. She said, I was told you enjoy snacking on these. I took them, placed a few in my mouth and thanked her. Her name is Mother Marzee O. Cannon of Warren Ohio. Mother Cannon, as I affectionately calls her became the Chairman of the Board of Women of Faith and Power Ministries, Inc... I love Mother Cannon and I pray that all her days are lived in peace and harmony.

Father, I thank you for all the reminders that you send me each day, to remind me of your love, and how much you care for me. In Jesus Name

There is in every true woman's heart
a spark of heavenly fire, which lies dormant
in the broad daylight of prosperity,
but which kindles up and beams
and blazes in the dark hour of adversity.
Washington Irving

We need to persevere so that
when we have done the will
of God, we will receive
what HE has promised.
Hebrews 10:36

I returned and saw under the sun that
The race is not to the swift,
Nor the battle to the strong,
Nor bread to the wise,
Nor riches to men of skill;
But time and chance happen to them all.
Ecclesiastes 9:11

God

grant me

the Serenity

to accept the things

I cannot change...

the Courage to

change the things

I can... and the

Wisdom to know

the difference.

The Oyster

When God created the oyster, He quaranteed him
complete economic and social security.
He said, "You will have a home built for you at the
bottom of the ocean, underneath the ocean mud, safe
and protected. You will have no worries for food, just
open your mouth and the food will flow in. Everything
will be taken care of for you. The oyster will not have
to go anywhere to live and prosper."

The Eagle

When God created the eagle, He quaranteed him
nothing. He said, " You will build your own
home, you will build it upon the highest mountain top.
There you can survey all, scream your defiance
For food you will range far and wide." The eagle was
quaranteed nothing!

The Penquins

There were twelve penquins in a family and they all
lived, traveled and slept together.
One day, the father figure, said to the mother, we need
to go the ocean and bath, and catch some fish
before the winter sets in. They agreed, and told the rest
of the family. The middle one was a little weak
from an infection, so they had to walk slower than usual
so the weak one did not get left behind. As they
were approaching the ocean, they noticed a fox sitting
on the bank. The father said to the family, we must
all stick together like glue, so this old fox wont have
none of us for dinner.

The family slowly merged into the ocean with the weak
one out front and the others swam closely behind. That
old fox remained on the ocean's bank licking his lips,
preparing for his dinner, but he had to devise a
plan, but he had none. So he watched and waited for one
of them to get seperated on their return. All the family
members stayed close as they had agreed. Many fish
was caught and their pouches was filled to capacity. The
weak member was also loaded to the gills. After they all
was nice and full, well fed and bathed, they made their
way back up and out of the ocean.

Old man fox was still on his perch, watching for a mistake to be made, however, no mistakes was made. The plan was followed to the letter. The old fox was confused, and angry, so he ran away with his tail between his legs hungry and defeated.

Lord, help your people to stand and work together so that none will perish....Amen

Present Thought

"It seems we have the tendency to move away from the present. It's as if this habit is built into our DNA. At the most basic level, we think all the time and this takes us away. I believe in fantasy as well as reality. One must be fully present having contact with the immediacy of our thoughts in order to experience reality. Fantasy is a totality of being lost in thought.."......Evangelist/Apostle Mary F.Simmons

Life is whatever we plan for it to be.

Our servant if written down on paper or even recorded;

Otherwise--- our friend.

Life responds to our outer most and sweetest emotions.

If we are uncertain; it reflects insecurity.

If we are excited----then joy reveals itself on every plane.

Life is precise!

It gives the accurate importance of our thoughts. Therefore, to master life, we must master thinking.

The only thing we have is what we have created.

The only time there is, is what you believe.

Here and eternity

Ah there is life beyond the grave

....

You are

Because I am that I am

I am as He Is

Because you are created in His Image and Likeness

You and I are heirs and joint heirs

You and I are now in His bosom

Here we can agree

All that the Lord has ordained and anointed for us to do is His Will...................

How can we escape such great Salvation

If we love Him

There is no excuse

Because all excuses was nailed to the cross

Can you handle that?

We are saved to be saved

All we have to do is endure until the end

No pain, No drama

Just believe

Nothing can seperate us from the love of God

Unless we allow it

Read the book of life.............

I thank the Most High
That this time is chosen for me.
I am the favored child of Yahweh
I made the only choice
Thank you Father for choosing me.
You are my choice..............

Perfection is contagious.

Having perfected myself in this

I go to perfect myself in whatsoever I desire

I am perfect in every state..............

If I am perfect

Then so are you.

For we only choose

What we are

Here and now.

St Matthew 5:48

You take the if out of my life................

Now what?

I took the if out of your life....................

Now what?

What if?

I don't remember..............

You see...................it never existed!

We need each other

To encourage our independence

You don't have to tell me

I see it in you

You don't have to show me

I feel it from you....................

After all

We are

Here and now

All there is.............

One Lord, One Faith, One Baptism

Tell it
Show it
No matter what
I know it

I am that I am

I am what you are
You are what I am
What is my image of me?
What is your image of me?

We can see now dimly, then face to face
What we are not familiar with
Can we?

I see your image of me

In my time of reflection

I see my image of me

In your response to my presence

I see what you see

Because I know who I am.

We will continue to evolve

We will become what we believe

We will have what we desire

We will do what we choose.

Choose this day whom you will serve

As for me and my house, we will serve the Lord.

Joshua 24:15

Our paths criss-cross

To become parallel

What have we brought for each other?

What we each ....ourselves possess

Thank you
Thank you me
Thank you God
We are one
Reflecting each other.

My presence upon you
Protects you at all times
Your presence upon me
Enhances my am........ness

Like consciousness
You bring me success.

Recent Lives

I've lived it before

It was not as I would heve wanted it to be

So now, I've been given a second opportunity to live again

This time, I have life in Messiah with no regrets

How about you?

Witnessing

Every believer, whether or not they speak of Christ is a witness..............Acts 1:8

Therefore, if you have the Spirit of God you are a witness

We all are witnesses spiritual or natural..................for the defense or for the prosecution.

Celebrations

Magical moments that nurture the soul, defines our culture

Thinkof the foot..............it is a celebration that we have two to dance with

Creation is a celebration of Yahweh's love for man kind.

What have you celebrated recently?

Eternal Journey

Man that is born of a woman has only a few days and they are full of trouble.................Job 14:1

For man is born for trouble...............Job 5:7

Because all his days, task is painful and grievious, even at night his mind does not rest.

Why is this happening?

Father, Mother, God

Father............... giver

Mother........... catcher

God................. producer of all

God can and is Father, Mother and Creator

Who may abide under His Wings?

Adam, Male, Female

The text of Genesis does not tell us the sexual orientation of Adam, therefore, this person could have been male or female.

We must not assume anything, muchless that this first human being was male, but the word for the first human was simply adam.

This human was not called ISH until ISHAH was taken out.

Thirty-two thousand women were called Adam in Numbers 31.

Who knew?

Sabbath

The Hour cometh, and now is, when the true worshippers shall worship the Father in Spirit and in truth; for the

Father seeks such to worship Him.....................St. John 4:23

Eye openers

Revelation 14:6-7

Isaiah 58:13-14

St. Matthew 11:28

Bald as the mountain tops are bald with a baldness full of grandeur

Because thou must not dream, thou need not despair

But each day brings its petty dust on soon-------- choked souls to fill

and we forget because we must, and not because we will.

I'm nobody! Who are you?

Are you nobody too?

Then there's a pair of us-----------don't tell!

They'd banish us you know.

How dreary to be somebody!

How public like a frog

To tell your name the live long day

To an admiring bog!

Emily Dickinson

Greatness is a spiritual condition

Woke up to say good morning Holy Spirit

How are you darling angels?

I love you dear Heavenly Father

Let's go and become greater.

Evangelist/Apostle Mary F. Simmons

Quotes

A woman's always younger than a man of equal years.

Best be yourself, imperial, plain and true.

God's gifts put man's best dreams to shame.

My son sets to rise again
MFS

A large brained woman and a big hearted man
...............can they co-exist together?
MFS

Ice runs cold,feet runs to mischief as water is to life.
MFS

A Riddle or Two

Little woman went out to milk her cow

Little boy followed, what did he hear?

Calf arrived and said Ma'am

Little boy surely published it

and today women are called Ma'am!

How charming

MFS

What did the can opener say to the can?

Open me!

MFS

Forward I am heavy, but backward I am not

What am I?

A whale

He has married many women, but has never been married.

Who am I?

A Celibate

How many of each clean animals did Mariam take on the boat?

Answer..

If there are ten eagles on a fence and the farmer shoots a fourth of them, how many are left?

Answer..

If you were at a campsite with a candle, a woodstove, some matches and fat wood, which would you start first?

Answer..

Believer's Corner

A sure cure

Three Pastors in the South were having lunch in a diner. One said "Ya know, since summer started I've been having trouble with bats in my loft and attic at church. I've tried everything...............noise, spray, cats........nothing seems to scare them away". Another said, "Yea, me too. I've got hundreds living in my belfry and in the nartex attic. I've even had the place fumigated, and they won't go away." The third said, "I baptized all mine, and made them members of the church.....................Haven't seen none back since!"

The Dead Church

A new Pastor in a small town spent the first days making house calls to each of the members, inviting them to the first service. The following Sabbath (Saturday) the church was all but empty. Accordingly, the Pastor placed a notice in the local newspapers, stating that, because the church was dead, it was everyone's duty to give it a decent burial. The funeral would be held the following Sunday afternoon.

Morbidly curious, a large crowd turned out for the "funeral." In front of the pulpit, they saw a closed coffin, covered in flowers. After the Pastor delivered the eulogy, he opened the coffin and invited the congregation to come forward and pay their final respects to their dead church.

Filled with curiosity as to what would represent the corpse of a "dead church" all the people eagerly lined up to look in the coffin then quickly turned away with a quilty sheepish look.

In the coffin, tilted at the correct angle was a large mirror. Anything dead ought to be buried!

St. Matthew 8:22

Satan----In--------Law

One bright Sabbath Morning, everyone in this little tiny Southern town got up early and went to Sabbath School at the local worship center. Before Sabbath School, the people was sitting in their seats. Suddenly, Satan appeared at the front of the church. Everyone started screaming and running for the exit, trampling each other in a frantic effort to get away from the evil one. Soon everyone was evacuated from the building, except for one elderly gentleman who sat calmly in his seat, not moving...............seemingly oblivious to the fact that God's ultimate enemy was in his presence.

Now this confused and irritated the devil, so he walked me?" So he walked up to the man and said," Don't you know who I am?" Yep, sure do, "the elderly man replied", Satan asked "Aren't you afraid of me?"

This time the man said, "Nope, sure ain't!" Satan,a little more perturbed at this, asked, "Why aren't you afraid of me?" The man calmly replied, "Been married to your sister for 56 years."

Gossip......Doing the Devil's Work for Him
We live in a nortoriously violent society! Under the
influence of Satan, people hurt, mame and kill
fellow humans with impurity. What about you? Do
you afflict injury upon your neighbors? Could you be
guilty of
murder? "How unthinkable!" You may answer.
"Never!"

Yet millions of seemingly harmless people hurt and even
kill their neighbors every day. Their instrument
of violence is not a steeley switch blade nor a silver
"Saturday night special" (an american term for a cheap
hand gun). It's the tongue!   "The hypocrite with his
tongue destroys his neighbor.........Proverbs 11:9
Whether the gossip is premediated or accidental,
murder is murder. And when one is dead, they are
dead. Yes, words
in the form of gossip can hurt you and other people.
However,gossip can be stopped! Let's learn how to
prevent this deadly crime. First, what is gossip? Many
people don't know. Many do know, but pretend they
don't. Many know, but don't care, they go right on
anyway, murdering others with their words. So let's
define this instrument of death.

What is Gossip?

Gossip accuses people. It charges others with wrong.
People love to talk about the alledged actions
of others. Does the following sound familar?
Did you hear what he did?
No tell me!"

"Well, just between you and me, he............" and on and on it goes.

Listen to what God says about gossiping accursers: "An ungodly man digs up evil, and it is on his lips like a burning fire"................Proverbs 16:27

What happens to the victim of accusations? These accursers, this lynch mob of tongues charge him, convict and condemn him to death! Accusation is deadly gossip.

Gossip slanders neighbor. It destroys a person's character or personal reputation. But beware! He who lives by the sword of slander shall die by the sword of slander. Almighty God warns, " Whoever secretly slanders his neighbor, him I will destroy"...........Psalm 101:5

Gossip talks indiscreetly. People who say just anything that comes into their minds spread gossip. They do not engage their minds before they engage their tongues. They do not evaluate what they are about to say or its effect on others. "A serpent may bite when it is not charmed; the blabber is no different"...........Ecclesiastes 10:11......In short, gossip is any communication that hurts people. "The words of a tale bearer are as wounds, and they go down into the innermost parts of the belly."...............Proverbs 18:8

What is the source?

Now you know what gossip is, but do you know where
it comes from? Whether you realize it or not, when you
gossip you are involved in an encounter with the realm
of evil spirits.   An encounter with the longest and vilest
tongue in the universe..................of satan the serpent.
Satan started gossip.   Jesus Christ said, "he was
a murderer from the beginning"...............St. John
8:44.   Satan probably used gossip to assassinate God
in the eyes of one third of the angels, caused them to
rebel..........Revelation12:4
Jesus also revealed that Satan is a lying slander: "For he
is a liar and the father of it..................St. John 8:44
Satan accuses both God and human beings today
through unsuspecting people. He is called the "accuser
of the brethren of God's begotten children in His
church................Revelation 12:10
Listen as Jude describes the gossiping nature of
Satan and his demons................with his people who
follow Satan's way: "Likewise also these dreamers
defile the flesh, reject authority, and speak evil of
dignitaries.   But these speak evil of whatever they do
not know or understand; and whatever they know
naturally, like brute beasts, in these things they corrupt
themselves............Jude 8-10. Yes Satan is the source of
gossip. Do not allow Satan to whisper in your ear

Gossip Addicts

People gossip for many...............all of them wrong reasons. For example, people of low self-esteem tend to gossip. They do not respect themselves, so they gossip about others and pull them down. This allows their egos to rise on the ruins of others. The gossiper experiences a temporary illusion of worth, but quickly descends even lower than before. He or she then yearns to gossip again,aching to experience another high. But deep down, they must continue to practice this devise so that they will feel good about themselves. This is only a temporary fix, because these people are addicts just as a drug addict, alcoholic, food , sex, or thrill seekers.

Frustration and boredom produces this type of behavior also, along with idleness wandering from house to house pretending to be your friend. People who are lazy tend to be engaged in the affairs of others. These people are relatives to the grave yard, they are never satisfied. The swan ehoes great discontent with this type of spirit and warns the believer to be on their guard at all times.

The cure for gossip

First realize how much God hates this type of behavior. Gossipping is a sin and it appears three times on God's "hit list" of the seven most abominable things He hates: (1). A lying tongue.........(2)..A false witness who speaks lies (3). sowing discord among the brethren (4) A proud look (5) hands that shed innocent blood (6)An heart that deviseth wicked imaginations (7) feet that be swift in running to mischief...........Proverbs 6: 17-19. This type of behavior is detrimental to the body of Christ and it must be stopped immediately. Our attitudes and behavior must be about building one another up, not about destroying one another. Repentenance must be preached in strength and power of the Holy Ghost with all rebuke and chastisement. The ones that are practicing and participating must be warned of God's impending judgement against such ones. Not only that, those that are strong must bear the infirmities of the weak, by teaching, counseling and using the authority that God has left to the church. We must not be cowards and children in our faith when it comes to this kind of behavior. Another important part of our gossip detection system is purity. The words must be pure. In our sick society, blasphemy and profanity almost have become proper etiquette. Their throat is an open tomb............ whose mouth is full of cursing (foriegn unknown carnal knowledge) and bitterness.........Romans 3: 13-14. God does not want His people listening to or spreading this filth around. We must keep our mouth filled with the pure word of God.

Love

Love isthe fulfillment of the Laws of God.......... without love we are as an empty wagon making a whole lot of noise and no one is paying any attention to us. With all of our knowledge, we must sure love at all times. No one wants to know how much we know, until they find out how much we care.

Love worketh no evil, it covers,hides, secure, protects and assures. Commandment Keepers must be Commandment Doers with a heart full of love and a mouth that is filled with praise. Our love must be first to the House Hold of Faith and then spread abroad. One must not be set in his or her on ways, rather ground and rooted in the ways of the Most High God. Our ways and our thoughts, must be the ways and thoughts of the Lord. We cannot even trust our own thoughts, they will and do lie to us continually. It is important to know the thoughts of God and walk in them at all times. Our love must not grow old or cold. Many people are different, we have to be adaptable as well as flexible when it comes to winning souls. A soul winner must be wise in word and deed.

Comfort Zones

It is oh so nice not to be challenged into doing somethings that are new and different. Like eating healthy and avoiding excessive weight. Let me tell you, I enoy good food and plenty of it, however, carrying the extra pounds around is no fun. It wears me out, not only physical, but emotional. So changes had to be made to get fit. Getting fit means eating smaller portions more often. The goal is not to be hungry, because, I have found, hunger will drive you to over eat, and we will feel guilty afterwards. This is a challenge for me and life style changes as well as life saving and prolonging ones life is on the line. Difficult choices has to be made as well as maintained, so I have decided to embrace the challenge. My goal is not to be skinny, rather to be fit for the journey. It does not make any sense to dig our graves with our teeth. These life saving changes has to be made if we want to live a long, healthy and prosperous lives. We have no one to blame except ourselves for our failures and successes.

Let's began with reprograming our minds. The mind is the most powerful organ in the pbody. Whatever we program our mind to do, the other members will follow. Plan to program your mind today just as you program your computer or your television to perform task. Breakfast is the most important meal of the day.

Here are a few tips for you to consider:

Fresh fruits with oatmeal and a little meat such as, turkey bacon, beef sausage or even a little left over fish from dinner.

Scrambled egg whites made into an omelet with onions, peppers, low fat cheeses, with whole wheat toast.

Remember, we are eating to live, not living to eat.

Do not fry foods, your body will love you for it.

Eat Like a King or Queen for breakfast and like a pauper for dinner.

Prepare oatmeal water over night for a wake up beverage by placing a little in some water over night and the next morning pouring the water and drinking it for maximum health and even taking a little with you for a thirst quencher.

Bake whole wheat breads and muffuins with nuts, such as walnuts, pecans etc.

Learn to be creative and think outside the box. Eat six small meals a day plus a few healthy snacks throughout to help you feel satisfied. There is no need to feel deprived or unsatisfied.

Choose some fun things to do in order to get a little exercise. All of us can move something.

Relax and have fun............enoy your life and be joyful.

Remember to be creative and think outside of the box.

We all have comfort zones where everything feels safe and familiar. We tend to not want to venture beyond it, however, if we allow ourselves to stay there we will not be challenged, experience personal growth, or learn new and exciting things or form new relationships. In other words, this will cause us to be stagnated. It is important to venture above our ankles, knees and get involved deeper which will allow us to swim in our challenging and witnessing. Then we can do head stands, and flips with vigor and ecstasy.

Quotes

A scholar who cherishes the love of comfort is not fit to
be deemed a scholar
Lao Tzu

We shall have no better conditions in the future if we
are satisfied with all those which we have at present
Thomas Edison

If you remain in your comfort zone you will not go any
further
Catherine Pulsifer

Comfort zones are most often expanded through
discomfort.......
Peter McWilliams

We cannot become what we want to be by remaining
what we are...
Max DePree

Nobody ever died of discomfort, yet living in the name
of comfort has killed more ideas, more opportunities,
more actions, and more growth than everything else
combined. Comfort kills.
T. Harv Eker

He has laid the foundation and opened up the way,
what more can He do.
The Late Great Dr. Chief Apostle S.P. Rawlings

My Comfort Zone

I used to have a comfort zone where I knew I wouldn't
fail. The same four
walls and busy work were really more like jail. I longed
so much to do the
things I'd never done before, but stayed inside my
comfort zone and paced the same old floor.
I said it didn't matter that I wasn't doing much. I said I
didn't care for things like commission checks
and such. I claimed to be so busy with the things inside
the zone, but deep inside I longed for something special of my own.
I couldn't let my life go by just watching others win. I
held my breath, I stepped
out side and let the change begin. I took a step and
with new strength I'd never felt before.
I kissed my comfort zone good bye, closed and locked
the door. If you are in a
comfort zone, afraid to venture out, remember that all
winners were at one time filled with doubt.
A step or two and words of praise can make your
dreams come true. Reach for
your future with a smile; success is there for you!

You can't miss what you never had!
I never had a comfort zone.
I never had time to learn
my comfort zone, muchless
to get comfortable. At an early
age my mother made sure I never
was afraid or shy about anything..
I would wake up when she called in the

late night to find my dad for mom. I
would walk the long dark roads from
my home to the speak easie's house.
My dog and friend Jack would accompany
me down the road to find dad.
My comfort zone has never been defined. I
am truly grateful to a loving and caring mother.

MFS

Wisdom

Wisdom is the principle thing, yet in all of our getting,
an understanding is the
ingredient that spins the wheel.
Wisdom is an acquired taste.............it must be sought
and persued.
Perseverance will get the job done ask Solomon
Persistence breaks done resistance.
Persistance cries and God's hears and answers.
Wisdom builds her house.
Want wisdom......keep and do the commandments
Deut. 4:6
Keep therefore and do them; (commandments) for
this is your wisdom and your understanding in the
sight of the nations.

We must set our hearts to seek wisdom with all
diligence.

Debra K. Carey

Marriage

Husband's cleve (cling) to your wives. Next to God, she
is your most important treasure.
Don't date her just to marry her, date her for a lifetime
of dates.
Marriage is a celebration of your life together, to
cherish, comfort, sanctify, romance, shield,
shelter and protect for as long as she lives.
The wedding night is a time to reflect on the events of
the day with joy and laughter. Often we
we feel the need to consummate the marrige on this
night however, this is the night to rejoice,
caress, and enjoy the memories of what God has joined
together. We have a life time for making
all of our dreams to be fulfilled, why rush it.
The chase is better than the catch................now that the
catch is in the boat, clebrate and enoy
the bounty. This is also a time to relax, romance and
appreciate each other as you prepare for a
life time of ecstasy with your life's partner.
Take it slow...........Solomon looked and saw that under
the sun, the race is not given to the swift,
nor the battle to the strong, for time and chance
happens to us all. Eccles. 9:11
Consider Song of Songs.............Solomon took precious
time and she with him to explore and...
enjoy every inch of thier bodies before consummating
the marriage. Anticipation is a powerful
fore play.

She may not be what you want or thought in the
beginning, and neither could you be what she
expected, however, with your love and patience, God
can and will bring to you exactly what you desire.
Treat her with care, love and devotion like the queen she
truly is, and she will treat you like the
king that you are. Make her feel pretty and secure, give
her no reason to ever question your...
love or committment. Allow her to be the center of
your life, and she will respect you and you,
will be known in the gates, men will envy and admire
your devotion to your bride.
I enjoy watching older couples that have weathered the
storms of life yet still clinging to each
other, living a life of savor and mystery with great
expectation and anticipation.
Husbands are never to leave their wives.............no
matter what.   If the wife is so unhappy and
miserable after all that he has done and provided, love,
shared and cared.........let her leave.
The husband is commanded by the Almighty God to
leave father and mother and cleve to his
wife..............Genesis 2:21-24.
God never changed His mind about this, and we must
obey the Lord in all things. There are
two immutable things that God cannot do: (1). He
can't lie (2).He will not change.................
Therefore, when you said.............in sickness, in
health...................rich or poorer until death do
us part............did you really mean it?   God was
listening and He is holding the both of you...
mutually responsible.

Children

Except the Lord build the house, they labour in vain
that build it: except the Lord keep
the city, the watchman waketh but in vain. It is vain for
you to rise up early, to sit up late, to eat the bread
of sorrows: for so he giveth his beloved sleep.
Lo, children are an heritage of the Lord: and the fruit
of the womb is His reward. As
arrows are in the hand of a mighty man; so are children
of the youth.
Happy is the man that hath his quiver full of them:
they shall not be ashamed, but...
they shall speak with the enemies in the gate.......Psalm
127

Children are the sweet desserts of your enduring passion
for each others.
They are an extension of your love and compassion to
the world.
Children are our gift to one another.
They are future kings, queens, presidents, lawyers,
doctors, poets, writers.
Our children will follow in our foot steps, President
Obama's and all of those
who has paved the way in this nation.
Support them, embrace them, punish them yes, most
importantly treasure
them and encourage them to be all that they can be and
let them know that

failure is not an option.
Our children will have their own personalities, dreams
and desire's, let us...
support and encourage them without criticisms.
Support them now and share in their victories as well as
their triumps later.

Philosophy

Use of reason and argument in seeking truth and
knowledge of reality, especially of
the causes and nature of things and of the principles
governing existence.

Branches of Philosphy

1. Metaphysics......Greek , ("after pysics") seeks to
   describe the ultimate nature of reality.

2. Epistemology......or theory of knowledge, is closely
associated with metaphysics, and considers how people
come to know what they know. It is the study of the
nature, source, and limits of understanding.

3. Logic.....is the branch of philosophy devoted to
   understanding and expressing the ...

rules of reasoning and inference. Logic originated with
Aristotle, who got it from God, and introduced the use
of variables as a tool for describing logical argument in
general terms.

4. Ethics................is the study of principles for proper
   human behavior. It is primarily concerned with
   establishing moral guidelines and debating their
   usefulness.

5. Aesthetics.......is somtimes counted as a fifth branch of philosophy. It is concerned.... with the nature and benefits of art, beauty, and other sensual experiences.

All good and perfect gifts comes from the Lord,,,,,,,,,,,,,,seek Him early and you will find Him and He will give you the disires of your heart.   If you are not blessed and prosperous, there is no one to blame but yourself.

One of the most wonderful places on earth.

Penn Center / York W. Bailey Museum

The Penn School was founded in 1862 by Laura Towne a native of Pittsburgh PA. Laura devoted thirty-eight years of her life to the colored people (African Americans) of St. Helena Island, South Carolina along with many others that dedicated and specialized in the education of the under priviledged. This is love personified, made personal. Love is not only loving those that you know, but reaching out to those that are without. Love is loving in the worst of times and under the worst circumstances. These men and women, first showed how much they cared. I have been cautioned all my life to show how much I care before I start sharing my educational experiences. Our Lord and Saviour Jesus Christ always showed how much He cared no matter what the need even on the cross with the condemned.

Education.............The thing that amazes me the most is that as slaves the people was not allowed to read or write, and no one was allowed to teach them during that time. Our fore parents came through that phase of their lives by the grace of God. However, once slavery was abolished by Abraham Lincoln, the President, they could pursue education. The Lord knew that His people was coming out of slavery............nevertheless it look time, because He had to prepare the heart and mind of President Lincoln. The Lord has no hands, feets, or no human parts, except

He prepares us and uses us to accomplish His will, and this takes time. The Lord prepared all the men and women for this task long before it happened, and they were obedient and willing to the call. The Lord knows the beginning from the end, and He has prepared away out for all of us, because, only He knows what will befall us.

The women was trained in domestics such as home making, cooking, cleaning, canning, raising children and other related work, mainly to be performed in the home. Midwives training was also a great asset in addtition to the much needed and appreciated assets that was taught to the women, so they could assist with local birth and care afterwards. Women helping women was and still is a wonderful and rewarding gift. There is nothing like resourcefulness and neighbor helping neighbors. This brings to life the commandment.............Love thy neighbor as thyself. Women was starter of fires in the morning. I can remeber my own mother rising early before anyone else to build a fire in the fire place and prepare breakfast, then she would wake dad, and help him get ready for the day. Then she would come and wake the children and get them ready for the day. Mom never sent us away without something warm and good in our bellies. Women could hunt, fish, trap and engage in the same activities as their counterparts. There was no government support, therefore, they had to be very crafty and resourceful even when it came to treating and caring for themselves, so they could be able to care for the family.

The men on the other hand where trained in building trades, maintenance, wood working and farming. Most of them were use to hard work with long hours and back breaking duties as they learned how to endure hardness as a good soldier unto the Lord. As you can imagine, there was not too many jobs available, so the men hunted, fished and planted the land that was given to them in order to feed their families. They lived off the land. I am in awe as I read the documented history of these our Patriachs and Matriachs as they depended on the Lord and carved out a great living. The Lord has always from the beginning prepared away for His people from the Garden of Eden. All we have to do is follow the master plan. Truly," He has laid the foundation and opened up the way, what more can He do." They were strong, and full of faith and power. Today, all of us have the same abilities and fortitudes if only we would embrace them without thinking that someone owes us a living. No one owes us nothing, but to love us. Our attitudes, persistent, perserverance and faith in the Lord esus Christ will prevail everytime. We are the head and not the tail, above only and not beneath.

Many great Patriach'a and Matriach's came from Penn School such as: Dr. York W. Bailey, whom the museum is named for. In 1906 he returned home to St. Helena Island as the only black doctor to serve his people with the assistance of nurses and midwives, who was trained to assist with the deliveries of babies and after care. Congressman Robert Smalls.........A Patriot's journey from slavery to capitol hill. This moving story is available @ Penn Center with a great many other historical collections. Mrs. Geraldine Simmons-White, a graduate of Penn School and secretary of the same, whom, I work with several times a week, went on to become a Registered Nurse and took care of countless veterans, came home to care for her mother and remained to help care for the people of the St. Helena Island community. Penn Center has a great collection of the fromer school relics and will take you down or bring back to your memories, things forgotten. I believe, every man, woman, and children should embrace this history and treasure it, share it, relish in it, brag about it, be proud of it, after all this is our inheritance. The Bible speaks of riding upon the high places of the earth and feeding us with the heritage of Jacob our Father......if this is not it, then I have missed something.

The Penn School closed in 1948 because of the State ran educational system and they no longer was able to compete, therefore, everyone was intergrated into public schools, where our fore parents continued to excel. Today, the York W. Bailey Museum show cases the history and struggles, along with victories that our fore parents treasured and sacrificed so we can enjoy them today. I am persuaded, with every success story there was a battle. One to be told. Our Matriach's and Patriach's endured the hardships as the Lord directed and strengthened them, so we won't, just as Jesus suffered on the cross and endured the beatings, markings, and humiliation for you and I. Today we are free and we have the freedom to become whatsoever we desire. Dr. Martin Luther King Jr. spent time at Penn Center working on "I have a dream". Today, I would hope and pray that each of you have a dream, and that you are instilling in your offsprings the importance and urgency of not only having a dream, but pursuing it and speaking of it as you share your plans to bring it to pass. Dr. Kings dream is a reality today and everyday we see branches of it coming into bloom and reality.

We must remember the past, please don't forget, however, don't allow it to be a road block to your future.

The word of God reminds us: Brethren, I count not myself to have apprehended: but this one thing I do, forgetting those things which are behind, and reaching forth unto those things which are before. We must never forget the past, however, the past can be a bridge to our future no matter what the race, condition or problem. I have a saying as I encourage our young people "Persistence breaks down resistance". All of my help comes from the Lord, I rely and depend on the word of God to get me through every situation, day, moment and decision. We must keep on knocking at the doors of life, just like our brethren in the scriptures and letters. It does not matter what time it is, knock with persistence and urgency, rather it be on heavens door or someone's else. Whatever or whoever is in the house, will eventually come to the door and see what the problem is. I find that people give up to soon and never realize that if I had kept on knocking, asking, believing, loving, caring, showing goodness and mercy as I waited, gold, silver or even platinum would have been mine. Children don't ever throw in the towel,,,,,,,,,,if you do, how do you know if you would have been victorious.

Life serves up many dishes, issues, challenges and triumps, yet, only the winner survives and lives to tell the story. In my own life, there has been all these and more, however, with the faith that was instilled in me at at very early age, I've learned how to trust and depend on the Lord. My elders has endured, and I am cut from the same cloth, their blood is running warm in my vain, therefore, I must press on to see what the end wil be. There is no quitting in me and I would hope that there is none in you. We must learn how to be creative and think outside the box in everything. As I travel across God's green earth, my goal and message is to teach everyone to find out where you came from and embrace it with courage and determination.

Now that I have said that, it is almost dinner time, and my mind has ventured to food which is one of my special delights, and I enjoy lots of good food. Let me share some of my favorites with you.

7Up Cake

> 3 cups self rising flour, presifted or use cake flour
>
> 5 eggs
>
> 3 sticks butter
>
> 1 cup 7 Up
>
> 2 cups sugar

Cream butter and sugar. Add eggs one at a time, blend each separately.

Preheat oven to 350 and bake until an inserted knife comes out clean.

Place dough in a bundt cake pan after you have sprayed it with pam or equivalent.

Pecan Pie

    3/4 cup sugar

    1 cup light karo syrup

    4 eggs slightly beaten

    4 Tbsp. butter or margarine

    1 tsp vanilla

    1 cup pecans chopped small

    Boil sugar and syrup 2 minutes

    Add butter and beaten eggs

    Beat well. Add pecans.

    Bake at 350 for 50 to 60 mins.

    Use a pie crust if desired

Corn Pudding

    1 can cream corn

    1 can whole kernel corn

    2 eggs

    1/4 cup can milk

    1/2 stick butter

    1 tsp. vanilla

    1/2 tsp. nutmeg

    1/2 tsp. cinnamon

    2 Tsp. brown sugar

    Place in a preheated oven 350

    Place in a pre greased pan and baked until golden brown

Potato Pone

> 5 lbs sweet potatoes
>
> 3/4 cup butter
>
> 3/4 cup sugar
>
> 1/2 cup milk/condensed
>
> 1 tsp. nutmeg
>
> 1 tsp. cinnamon
>
> 1 tsp. ginger
>
> 3/4 cup flour
>
> 1/4 cup grated orange or lemon peel

Mix all ingredients and cook on top of stove in a heavy iron skillet

Put in baking pan, bake at 350 for 20 mins.

French Toast

    2 eggs beaten

    1 cup milk

    1 Tsp. sugar

    2 tsp. cinnamon

    1/2 tsp. nutmeg

    a dash of ginger

Mix sugar, nutmeg, cinnamon and sugar together, add milk, mix well. Dip bread on both side .

Put in hot greased skillet.

Brown on both sides

Sprinkle with a little powdered sugar and fresh fruit.

Ohio Coffee Bread

2 cups complete buttermilk pancake mix

1/2 tsp. ground cinnamon

1/2 tsp. ground ginger

2/3 cup milk

1/3 cup sugar

1 cup molasses

2 Tsp. butter

In a bowl combine pancake mix, cinnamon, and ginger until well mixed. Remove 1/3 cup of the mix; set aside. Combine milk and molasses; add to dry mixture. Stir just until moistened. Do not over mix. Turn into a greased 9 inch pie plate. In a small bowl combine the reserved pancake mix and sugar. Cut in butter until mixture resembles coarse crumbs. Sprinkle ove batter. Bake in a 350 degree oven about 25 minutes or until a tooth pick comes out clean. Serve warm or cool.

Green Salad

Shredded or chopped

Lettuce

Cabbage

green, yellow, and red bell peppers

tomatoes

cheeses

egg plant

broccoli

Wash vegetables well

Top with your favorite cheeses

Dressings

A drissle of honey

and

Serve them with crackers and peanut butter

Add a little meat if desired

Meats are a small favorite of mine, but they must be grass fed and cooked to perfection. In my book "Divine Healing + Divine Health = A Divine Life, I explain the procedure for optimum health and longevity God's way. Not only must it be free from chemicals, it must be fed the right ingredients, beacuse whatever the choice you choose, remember, it goes into your blood stream and enters the rest of your body. We would prefer, you make an informed decision so you can live a long and helathy life free of diseases and sicknesses. Therefore, choose wisely when it comes to meat products.

The Loves Of My Life

Deuteronomy 6:4-6
Sh'ma Yisra'el Adonai Eloheinu, Adonai Ekhad--Hear,
O Israel, The Lord
Our God Is One.
I Love The Lord With All My Being
I Love Myself

Therefore, I Love My Neighbors
And
Others As I Love Myself
These verses are called the Shema meaning to hear.
One
Complete Unity Or Togetherness
Oneness
One Lord
Love Thy God
Love Thyself
Love Thy Neighbor
Do Unto Others As You Would Have Them Do Unto
You
Love is the motive behind our relationship to God.
This Is The First And Great Commandment
St. Matthew 22:38
God Has No Higher Commandment Than Love
Love Fulfills The Law Of God
The Law Is Summed Up In One Word....Love
If.................A Qualifier
If.............Eye Opener

If You Love Me Keep My Commandments
St. John 14:15
And thou shalt love the Lord thy God with all thine
heart, and with all thy soul,
and with all thy might.
We cannot love anyone or anything properly unless we
fall in love with the Lord
first and put Him first in our lives.   I have seen people
who claim to love someone else, when they don't
even love themselves. Let us turn the spot light on
ourselves and seek the face of God in order to get a right
prospective and live a life of happiness and prosperity. I
love the Lord and His Saints and all those that the Lord
bless to be the keepers of His door.   I come alive at the
mention of the Lord and look forward to spending an
eternity in His Kingdom as I reign and rule with Him
throughout the ages.

The Holy Names Of The Father Almighty God

1. Elohim.....the ordinary Hebrew name.....I Samuel 28:13, Psalm 82:1, St. John 10:34

2. EL...The strong one......Genesis 31:13, Genesis 20:5

3. EL-Bethel......God of Bethel.....EL Ganna....Genesis 28:19, Genesis 31:13

4. Elshaddai.......The Almighty.....Genesis 17:1, Genesis 28:3, Numbers 24:4

5. EL ELYon.......Most High God......Genesis 14:18, Psalm 82:6, St Luke 1:32

6. Adonai.....Lord....Dependence....Acts 16:17, Acts 7:17, Acts 18:12, St Mark 5:7

7. Yahweh....Jahweh....Genesis 4:25, Exodus 6:20, St John 5:26, Exodus 3:10

8. Jah.......if there was no J, there would be no Jesus (Yahshua....Salvation).....Acts 4:12 Exodus 15:2, Psalm 68:4, Isaiah 11:2, Isaiah 26:4, Genesis 2:4-Genesis 3:22, Amos 5:27

9. Jahweh....Tsebaoth......Isaiah 19, Isaiah 63, Psalm 84:1

10. Jehovah Jireh......My Provider....Genesis 22:14

11. Jehovah Sees.......St. John 11:34

12. Jehovah Nissi....God is my banner....Exodus 17:15

13. Jehovah Shalom......Judges 6:24   God is my peace

14. Jehovah Shammah... God is there.....Ezekiel 48:35, Isaiah 60:14, Isaiah 6:22, Rev. 21:21

15. Jehovah Tsidkenu......Our Righteousness.....Jeremiah 23:6, Jeremiah 33:15

Why Does The Swan Echoe?

The swan echoes for all those that does not have a voice, has not made their moderation known unto the Lord. Those that are still living beneath there abilities, hiding behind something or someone. Their lights are still hiding under a bushel. Those who have refused to claim and walk in their inheritance. Those who have allowed the prison, ghettos, oppression, depression, manipulators, evil doers, and all manner of opposition to hinder and be in them to the point where fear has became their best friend. You have refused to rise up and say enough is enough. Those who are living in poverty and have blamed it on society, family, circumstances or environment. Life is just passing you by. I drive by many cemetaries and I see so many lost opportunities, that it makes me ill. Lost opportunities to have written books, poems, poetry, newsletters, quotes, motivational, inspirational and dynamic letters of marketing, advertising and sermons of hope, dreams, restoration and only God knows what else.

The swan desires that none perish just as the Lord does, yet we realize that some of you will continually let the good that the Lord has placed in you pass on over to some one else. The Lord designed and made us all for a purpose. Why not ask Him, what is your purpose in life. Just because you were born in the ghetto, does not allow the ghetto to be in you...that is your call. We can blame no one for our missed opportunities. We must be prepared when an opportunity presents itself...that is why

117

they call it luck.   Preparedness meets an opportunity...
this is what they call LUCK!

The Swan echoes continually for those who would
rather sit around and complain, rather than, thinking
outside of the box, getting involved, wiriting down on
paper, your plan for a successful life and using the word
of God as your role model and not only coming up to
the plate, but coming up, full of wisdom, knowledge and
understanding and knocking the ball out of the park. We
must do our home work on the companies, that we are
looking to work for. It impresses me to no end, to have a
young person, walk into my office, shake my hands, while
looking into my eyes, and speaking expressly to me about
me and about my accomplishments. Don't you think,
your future employer would be so impressed with you and
your presentation, that he or she will hire you right on the
spot. We must not only, brush our teeth, comb our hair,
press our clothe, shine our shoes, but we must impress
with a smile that is infectious with no return. Success is
worn at all times. Even if you don't have a job, act like
you do everyday. Don't allow life to pass you by............
God has ordained you for greatness....Do Not Settle For
Less! We would like for you to build up your most holy
faith in the word of the Lord and stay there until Jesus
comes, this is why I write the way I do, not for my sake,
but for yours.......GO OUT AND MAKE ME HAPPY
TODAY!

**Other Books, Tapes, & DVD's That Will Inspire
And Motivate You that the Lord has
blessed me to write, record or produce.**

Why The Swan Sings
The Old Woman And The River
Sarah's Story
Divine Healing + Divine Health = A Divine Life
A Documentary of The Early Life Of Evangelist /
Apostle Mary F. Simmons
Creature's Clean & Unclean
In The Time Of Need
A Designated Diet
Healing Is Yours For The Asking
Live In Portsmouth Ohio Pastor Lattimore & The
Saints
Women of Faith and Power Ministries, Inc., First
Dinner
Educational Messages
Radio Broadcasts
Valuable Information In Time of Need
If Thou Canst Believe
History of the Church
Faith Without Works
Be Content
A Calendar Comparison
Mutt & Jeff
WFPM Vision
WFPM Luncheon
New Home
Questions & Answers
In The Time Of Trouble

Help From Hidden Hands
Out Of Prison To Reign
Who Is The Holy Spirit?
Set The Captives Free.....6 tape series (90 mins. each)
Doctrine of Spiritual Gifts
A Two Kind Of Love
Why The Swan Sings Series (60 mins. each)buy the
books and tapes are free
Faith Worketh By Love
Unfulfilled............Women's Conference
Sabbath Morning Sacrifice
My Praise For His Glory......3 Tape Series
Behold How Good
Prayers Of The Forgiven with Poetry & Poems
From Clutter To Contentment
When Grace Has You In His Grip
Security In The Blood Of Jesus
Why Aren't Our Prayers Answered Today?
Forty Reasons ....God's Law Or Man's
Are You Praying In Details?
The Four Horses Of The Apocalypse
And Many Many More Ministerial Resources
Email Evangelist/Apostle @Simmmary@yahoo.com for
prices and info.

Why The Swan Sings Memorable
www.zazzle.com
T-Shirts
Mugs
Calendar
Tote Bags
Chanukah Cards

Why The Swan Sings Calendars
www.lulu.com

amazon.com

Follow The Evangelist Mary F. Simmons
twitter.com

facebook.com

essence.com

ryze.com

BET.com

Newsletter & Updates Website
http://www.womenoffaithandpowermi.injesus.com

Travel & Employment

www.simsvacationtravel.biz

Click On Test Drive, Training, Family Vacations and Opportunities

Call... Vondalyn Simmons   843 986 0341 for further details

Brother Willie Kirkland

Photographer & Videographer

843 726 4107

History & Culture

www.penncenter.com

Tours

The Spirit Of Old Beaufort
843 525 0459

Revivals, Crusades, Motivational, Inspiration Speakers
843 683 2026
Womenoffaithandpower@injesus.com

Ghost writers/ Help With Writing & Publishing
Simmmary@yahoo.com

We Need Financial Backers To Help Us Produce
Plays & Launch Our Ministry
Womenoffaithandpower@yahoo.com

Pre-Paid Legal Services, Inc.
Alexander Ravenel, II & Bishka Ravenel
ravenel83@predaidlegal.com
843 412 3242

People I Admire

Gloria J. Campbell, BFF
President & First Lady Obama
President & Secretary of State William Jefferson &
Hillary Rodham Clinton
Former Secretary of State Ms. C Rice
Pastor Geraldine Simmons
Bishop/Apostle Larry Owens
Rev. Jessie Jackson
Elect Lady Mary Rawlings
Evangelist Stella Taylor
Chief Apostle & Elect Lady James E. Embry
Elect Lady Sandra Lattimore
Shirley Ceasar
Juanita Bynum
Joel Osteen & Family
Susie Mae Simmons
Eugene & Loy Simmons
Elizabeth Carney
Oprah Winfrey
Whoopi Goldberg
Mary I. Mack
The Members of The House of God
The Chabad Congregations
Jews For Jesus
Commandment Keepers
Jerome Simmons
Darlene D. Simmons
Philip Q Simmons

Lynn Markovich Bryant author of I'm Black And I'm
Proud
Karen   Ward
Mrs. Julia Simmons
Ms. Rosalyn Browne
And All People Who Take A Stand In Life And
Proclaim Their Beliefs

Special Thanks Too:

Pastor Geraldine Simmons and Congregation for allowing me the time and opportunity to share my life and love with the multitude of fans and admirers on the Sabbath Day. It is a joy to share my life with you. My mother Susie Mae Simmons, who still laughs at my humor and still calls me Frances. I love you for all time Mom, you have and will always be my girl. My co-workers, friends, supporters and cheer leaders, I love you one and all. The Boys & Girls Club of Jasper County, I embrace you all, therefore, let's make many things happen this coming year so we can be a light to Jasper and surrounding communities. My brother Eugene and Loy Simmons, I am truly indebted to you for the use of your car. Without it, I don't know what I will have done. You will be well rewarded just you wait and see. My son Philip Q., I miss you so much, when will I see your face again?

Resources & Helps

The Holy Bible, King James & English Version
The Liberty Bible Commentary
The New YorK Times Guide To Essential Knowledge
Oxford Pocket Dictionary and Thesaurus
The Internet
Bird Lovers
The Columbia Encylopedia
The Late Great Dr. Kenneth Hagin Sr.

Father, I thank you for the wisdom, knowledge and understanding that you have given me with the ability to articulate my words and actions. Thank you for the hills, mountains and valleys that you have allowed me to experience during this time of research and writing. It has not been easy, yet, you inspired and motivated me to do my very best and to bring about another master piece so your people will be able to say, I am without excuse once again," For You Have Laid The Foundation And Opened Up The Way What More Can You Do?" Thank You Father In Jesus Name for using such a wretch as I......
Amen

Please take a little time out and pray the prayer of Colossians 3:12-17 for me and my staff.

Thank You and may God richly bless you and your family.

Your Servant
Evangelist/Apostle Mary F. Simmons
Simmmary@yahoo.com
Womenoffaithandpowermi.injesus.com

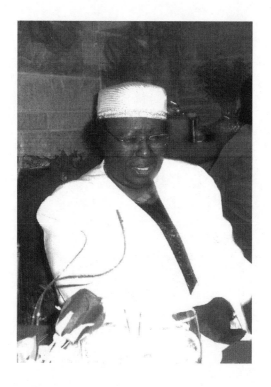

Evangelist/Apostle Mary F. Simmons is a well organized woman with the Spirit of God living, breathing, walking and moving in her. She has been anointed and ordained to preach, teach, write, administer all the works and services of the Lord. Mary is endowed with a seven fold ministry and she loves to be used of the Lord and to be a blessing to His people.

Manufactured By: RR Donnelley
Breinigsville, PA USA
February, 2011